CONTENTS

No-Cost Ways to Looking Younger

Eat Your Way to Weight Loss

Your Dietary BFF's

Things You Don't Usually Think About

When Less is More

ACKNOWLEDGEMENTS

I would like to thank my colleagues, relatives and friends who generously contributed their time, knowledge and experience to bring this book to life. Special "arigato" to Dr. Kiyoko Kato, Dr. Satoko Katayama, and Dr. Charlie Brannon, my medical and science advisors; and to Lin Sakai, TC Swartz and my Mirai Clinical family who help me grow each day.

INTRODUCTION

Did you know that Japanese women are healthier, thinner, younger-looking, and live longer than any other women in the world? It's a bold statement, but it's true.

In this book, I'm going to let you in on my country's most coveted beauty and health secrets so you, too, can enjoy the same youthful benefits that those in my culture have known for centuries. These secrets include things that people outside of Japan would never even talk about!

Not surprisingly, as a Westernized diet and more modern lifestyle have gained popularity in Japan, researchers have noticed an increasing number of healthcare issues in the elderly; yet, despite these influences, there is still a significant gap between the life expectancy of a Japanese woman (86) and an American women (81)*. The obese population in Japan is 3% while in America it is 34%**. Breast-cancer rates (one-in-eight among US women) are only one-in-20 among the Japanese***; a significant difference that's attributed to the unique way we eat and take care of our bodies.

I was born and raised in Hokkaido, the northern-most island--known for the purity of its waters and the beauty of its women, the majority of whom have clear, supple, translucent skin. This is a culture that reveres nature and, over the centuries, has learned to harness its remarkable preventive and healing powers. It's a culture where many elders live healthfully into their 90s, without heart disease or cancer; where our children happily drink green tea and eat fresh vegetables from a very young age.

I became acutely aware of the differences between the Japanese and Western lifestyles when I was 20 years old and lived as an exchange student with a family in Portland, OR. Everything—including the food—was so new and exciting, that I took it all in with great gusto. I also took in about 10 extra pounds from all the cheeseburgers, fries, pasta, candy, and soda that I ingested on my two-week visit. Friends and family back home were shocked at my appearance when I got off the plane; in addition to being heavier than I'd ever been, my skin had also taken a turn for the worse. In that defining moment, I realized what you eat and how you live plays an even bigger role in health and beauty than pure genetics.

It was a big, fat lesson for me. Literally.

Shortly thereafter, I began to religiously adopt the wisdom my mother had preached at me my whole life: eat carefully and nutritiously, maintain good posture, and protect your skin from the sun at all times. As my appearance changed for the better, so did my confidence level; and it wasn't long before I decided to make the field of anti-aging my mission—and profession—in life.

I got an M.B.A. at a university in Hong Kong and I studied for my international beauty license. I moved to the US, where I was shocked to learn that women spend hundreds of unnecessary dollars on synthetic skincare products that deliver empty promises, and actually age you in the long run.

Even as a US resident—with all the temptations of those cheeseburgers looming!—I practice what I preach. I exercise; I do some pretty "out-there" health and beauty rituals; I eat small portions of healthy, flavorful food in tremendous variety; and I zealously guard my skin from the sun. (Want to know how zealously? I was actually stopped by the police for wearing a haz-mat helmet on one of my daily walks!)

In this book, you will learn all my secrets, which are based on a holistic lifestyle that extends far beyond the reach of products you buy in a store. Adapting and adjusting to these Japanese principles may take some time—and some patience—but I promise you, the results will be worth it.

* List of countries by life expectancy by the United Nations (2005-2010)
** Estimated Obesity (BMI ≥ 30 kg/m²) Prevalence, Females, Aged 15+OECD, Health at a Glance 2009
*** Pink Ribbon, information in 2010

Here Comes the Sun:
Preparing Your First Line of Defense

1. UV RAYS CAUSE 80% OF YOUR SKIN DAMAGE

We've all heard the warnings about the dangers of the sun and its proven connection to wrinkles, sun spots, and melanoma. But dermatologists say 80 percent of skin aging is caused by UV rays. And no matter how much the sales people, magazine articles, and TV infomercials tell you otherwise, no sunscreen on the market actually blocks the sun completely. In fact, did you know that the FDA recently made a decision to ban the word "block" from being used on sun-protection products? So while manufacturers can talk up the yin yang about the importance of frequent and plentiful applications of high-level sunscreen, some damaging rays will always manage to seep through, regardless of how many times you diligently reapply. (This is discussed further in the next chapter.)

The Japanese have shared this perspective for a long time—which is why, if you spend any time in my country, you're likely to see some pretty "radical" strategies to stave off the sun. And I'm not just talking about wearing a cute hat or visor; the Japanese take it to the extremes. You might see:

- **Umbrellas** made with UV-protective fabric (you can even buy a special gizmo that attaches the umbrella to your bike)
- Up-to-the-elbow **gloves**
- Helmet-like **face coverings**
- **Laundry detergent** with built-in sunscreen claiming that the more you wash, the more protection will be delivered to your clothing
- UV **sun "sensors"** that attach to your cell phone or key ring (they change color when the exposure increases)

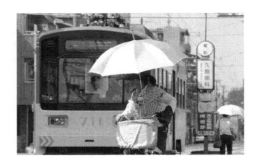

Look Ma! No hands! (And no wrinkles, either.)

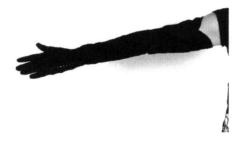

Treat your skin to opera-length gloves—no special occasion needed.

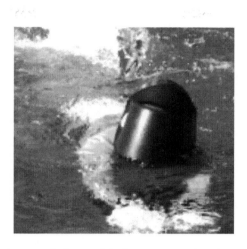

This haz-mat helmet might be extreme—but don't take
thorough face- and head-covering for granted.

The idea of toting a giant umbrella to your next outdoor concert isn't
sounding so weird anymore, is it?

The items are actually available outside of Japan, too.   Go ahead and
Google these product.

.

2. UV-AGING AND UV-BURNING

But back to those SPF's: the only way to understand the whole sunscreen puzzle is to learn what that big ball of fire in the sky actually does to your skin when you walk outside. Without getting too technical, let me give you a quick explanation:

The sun is shining; you're dying to feel the warmth on your skin, so you grab your towel and hit the beach. That wonderful sensation you feel? It's made up of UVB and UVA rays; think of the former as powerful-but-superficial rays...the ones that only get as far as the outer layer of the epidermis, and cause the lobster look we commonly refer to as "sunburn". They're damaging, but on an external level. Let's remember this as UV Burning.

UVA rays, on the other hand, are far more destructive: they can penetrate through glass (which is why pilots, who sit in front of big cockpit windows, are frequently diagnosed with melanoma), and penetrate deep into the basal layer of the epidermis, where skin cancers begin. Let's remember this as UV Aging. Tanning machines use UV Aging rays, so don't be fooled when tanning-salon employees tell you that their beds only use the "safe" UVA rays to work their magic.

In an effort to protect you as much as humanly possible, manufacturers now voluntarily offer "broad spectrum" sunscreens, which mean they help shield against both UVB and UVA rays. In Japan, every sunscreen must offer UVB and UVA protection, but this is not yet required by the FDA in the US. Japan takes the whole business a step further; they actually categorize the amount of UVA protection in every sunscreen product. PA+++ is the highest strength on the market.

Now let's talk about those letters and numbers you see on the bottles. First, SPF stands for "sun protection factor"—or, the amount of time you can stay in the sun without getting burned. (The Japanese would say none!) The higher the number, the longer they claim to protect you—but only from UV Burning not UV Aging. There's actually minimal need to focus on the number. Instead, direct your attention to how much of that lotion, spray, or cream you apply to your skin, and how frequently you do it. In actuality, a broad spectrum SPF 15, applied thickly and liberally over a three-hour period, will protect you from the sun far better than one squirt of a broad spectrum SPF 50. Add sunscreen-packed foundation and moisturizer to the mix and you'll be in even better shape.

But frankly, a haz-mat suit beats SPF hands down.

3. DON'T EAT LEMONS IN THE MORNING, BUT DO EAT TOMATOES AT NIGHT

Vegetables and fruits are obviously good for you, but did you know that some of them should be eaten at specific times?

Avoid eating these fruits and vegetables during the day: lemons, oranges, grapefruit, celery, parsley, potatoes, and eggplant.

Why? They include a substance called Psolaren that is known to absorb UV rays. Ingested psoralen makes your skin more sensitive to UV rays, which causes 80% of skin aging. But, psoralen breaks down in 8 hours, therefore it's fine to eat those fruits and vegetables at night.

This warning applies to cosmetics, too. If your moisturizer or serum includes extracts from the vegetables and fruits discussed above, for example, lemon (Citrus Medica Limonum - lemon oil), you are at risk of absorbing more skin-unfriendly UV rays. Retinol also has the same UV-absorption effect as psolaren. Cosmetics with these ingredients should not be used during the day, and only at night.

One vegetable that you should definitely eat at night is the tomato, which contains the powerful antioxidant lycopene offering many benefits for your body and skin. Lycopene has been known to help:

- Prevent skin damage from UV or any other oxidized stress
- Fight cancer
- Keep your cells strong and rejuvenated

Lycopene travels from the small intestine to your skin cells in 6-8 hours. So, by the time you're up and ready to go outdoors, the antioxidants from the lycopene will be ready to protect your skin from harmful UV rays.

Cooking tip: heating and mixing the tomato with oil maximizes absorption (bioavailability) into your system. Who knew your mom's favorite pasta sauce recipe was so good for you?

4. JACKIE O'S AND SUNCARE

Just as UV rays can damage your skin, they can damage your eyes. In fact, after just several unprotected hours in the sun, your eyes can become inflamed, red, even swollen and sore. (Need proof? Ever played volleyball at the beach on a bright day without your sunglasses?) As soon as that inflammation kicks in, it triggers a message to your pituitary gland that says, "Please create more melanin in the body to protect those eyeballs!" And now, just like those cool, photo-chromic lenses that darken the minute you go outside, you've got the body producing extra pigment to protect the skin from the sun's dangerous rays.*

That's great, right? Not so much...because it results in unsightly dark spots and freckles on everything from your cheeks to your chest to your hands. Even worse than unattractive skin, those UV rays can actually damage your eyes, leading to conditions such as cataracts or keratitis (inflammation of the cornea).

You're probably reaching for your sunglasses about now, so let's make sure you're choosing the right ones....

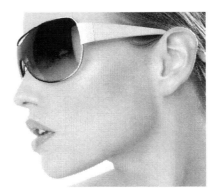

- **Go for the Jackie O's:** She may have been a style icon, but apparently she knew a thing or two about taking care of her eyes, too, since bigger is better when it comes to sunglass protection. Pay special attention to the sides, where light often sneaks in, and select a pair that covers as much of your temples as possible.

- **Look for dual coverage:** High-quality sunglasses will offer both UVA and UVB protection. Always check labels before you buy.

- **Avoid the dark side:** Though it may seem counter-intuitive, super-dark lenses force your pupils to open wide, and that lets in more light...and more of those UV rays to boot. You'll know you've got the right pair if people can actually see a bit of your eyes through the lenses. And if you just can't let go of your sexy blackout shades, please save them for Hollywood premieres or the front row of Fashion Week.

- **Make good contact:** If you wear contact lenses, look for a brand that features UV protection; your optometrist or ophthalmologist can help you find the proper pair.

* Keiichi Hiramoto and Masayasu Inoue of Osaka City University Medical School in Japan 2001

5. THE VITAMIN D DILEMMA

You might be wondering about Vitamin D, that vital nutrient for bone strength and immune system support. The dilemma: your body naturally produces Vitamin D when your skin is exposed to the sun, but applying sunscreen reduces its absorption. In addition, the sun induces the production of serotonin, which makes you feel happier, aids in resetting your biological clock, and helps to offset jet lag. So, what should you do?

First, keep in mind the negative affects of UV Aging and UV Burning rays, and exercise caution whenever you are exposed to the sun.

Second, add to your diet foods rich in Vitamin D such as salmon, mackerel, sardines, herring, cod liver oil, milk, eggs, and soymilk, plus a Vitamin D supplement. (Because of Japan's balanced diets, Vitamin D deficiencies are not as big a concern as they are in the USA.)

If you care about your skin's health but still want to sun-bathe, avoid exposing your face. Let the sun shine on normally shielded areas like your back, stomach, or thighs.

By the way, Vitamin D is synthesized only from UV Burning. Even if you are exposed to sunlight through a window, you won't get Vitamin D because the window shields off UVB. Unfortunately, it does not shield from UV Aging so do take the necessary precaution.

Is Your Skin Care Regimen Aging You?

6. THE BEST SKIN CARE CREAM
IN THE WORLD…

…is your skin's own natural moisture barrier.

Yes, you are born with the best skin care cream that Mother Nature can provide.

Your skin's natural moisture barrier is comprised of natural oils and sweat glands that defend against the culprits of aging such as dehydration, UVA and UVB rays, environmental pollution, cold temperatures, and even heavy makeup. Therefore, to maintain hydrated and healthy skin, it's critical to protect your natural oil barrier as much as possible by following the best skincare practices outlined in the next chapters.

Coupled with protecting the skin's natural barriers, is boosting your skin's natural rejuvenation cycle. The turnover rate for a single skin cell in a healthy, young person is approximately 28 days. That's how long it takes for a new cell to grow on the inside and emerge as fresh skin, causing the old, dead cells to naturally slough away. Because each cell is on a different cycle, it takes about 3 months for your body to go through a complete rejuvenation cycle. Unfortunately, the sloughing process slows down with age (e.g., the turnover rate for each cell on a 40-year-old might be about 40 days); those dead skin cells start accumulating and piling up on top of each other, resulting in a rough, dull complexion. Good exfoliation products can speed up the sloughing process…but certainly not in a day or two. Your goal to maintain youthful looking skin, then, is to stay as close to the 28-day rejuvenation process as possible. The following chapters will show you how..

7. INGREDIENTS YOU SHOULD AVOID

The first step towards achieving a 28-day rejuvenation cycle is to read the labels on cosmetics jars, and know what to avoid. Just as you (hopefully) read the labels of every food you put into your body, it's important to read the labels of products you apply to your skin.

These days, it's almost impossible to avoid seeing ads for skincare products that make some pretty significant claims. But just because the newest, hottest, most high-tech moisturizer on the store shelf advertises its instant wrinkle-busting powers, doesn't mean you should believe the hype. In fact, if a product tells you that using it will cause wrinkles to disappear instantly (or even in a matter of days), please keep walking—it's simply not true.

Manufacturers work very hard to create the most sophisticated skincare products possible; but not every ingredient works to your advantage. And when you see ingredients on face serums, moisturizers, washes and shampoos like:

- Cocamidopropyl betaine
- Polyethylene glycol (PEG)
- Sodium lauryl sulfate
- Sodium laureth sulfate

...put the item back on the shelf! These are known as synthetic surfactants; essentially, the workhorse ingredients in cleansers that go deep into your skin, emulsifying (or, breaking up and liquefying) dirt so that it can be loosened and removed. They are used because they are inexpensive and plentiful for manufacturers to use.

Synthetic surfactants are used in anti-aging moisturizers by breaking through the skin's barriers and enabling its active ingredients to penetrate deeper. However, by breaking the skin's natural barriers, these surfactants are damaging the skin's ability to keep moisture inside. By so doing, "anti aging" products with these synthetic surfactants are actually slowing down the skin's natural rejuvenation cycle and accelerating aging! And then they, fill the broken barrier with synthetic polymer, to leave the skin soft and smooth. But is it safe to do such unbiological stuff? You have to keep using such synthetics forever. For example, think about artificial sweeteners. We know that the artificial sweetener is not safe, but if you keep taking it, you get more addicted to the sweetness and keep taking more and more for the rest of your life. Such a vicious cycle.

Use products with these harsh ingredients too often and you'll find your skin to be drier and far more sensitive over the long haul. (Need more convincing? Some cleansing products contain as much as 30 percent synthetic surfactants, which is roughly the same level you'll find in dishwashing detergents!)

A better option: gentler products—such as the Mirai Clinical Purifying Face and Body Serums—designed specifically not to break your natural skin barrier, and effective for your face and entire body.

There's more.

Synthetic preservatives are used for obvious business reasons. Skin care and cosmetic products need a reasonably long shelf life and remain stable during hot summers, and under hot retail store lights. While good for business reasons, they are not good for your skin as they also damage the skin's natural moisture barrier. So, you might look for products that, like foods, have an expiration date or airless container, which means they have less preservatives than those with no expiration dates.

Now we get to those ingredients known as synthetic polymers, ingredients that cling to the skin and are frequently used to help produce a smoother appearance by absorbing water. Newsflash: synthetic polymers are also used in clear, plastic food wrap and diapers; but they're difficult to rinse off the skin (hence, the word "cling wrap"), and known to kill off good bacteria, thereby damaging your skin's delicate balance.

So, when you see words such as:

- Dimethicone
- Carbomer
- Acrylamide

......put the product back on the shelf and walk away.

Sometimes, manufacturers hide behind industry lingo to disguise harsh ingredients: For example, the words, *for professional use only* allow the manufacturer to avoid listing certain harmful chemicals on their ingredient list. Use of the word, *hypo-allergenic*, which makes something *sound* mild and skin-friendly, isn't actually regulated by the FDA; you'll see it used on a whole host of products that may, in fact, be less gentle than you think. Keep in mind that cosmetics and skin care products are not strictly regulated by the FDA, as are the food and pharmaceutical industries. So the well being of your naturally beautiful skin depends on your being your own well-informed consumer advocate.

8. ALL NATURAL IS NOT ALWAYS GOOD

Here's the problem with the phrase, "all natural": Unless you're talking about a product made entirely of home-grown, perishable ingredients (a sugar scrub, say, or an oatmeal mask), the term natural doesn't necessarily mean good for your skin.

Remember Chapter 3 about lemons, oranges, or grapefruit? While they are wonderfully healthy natural fruits, they contain psoralen, a substance that makes you extra-susceptible to UV rays and sun damage whether they are ingested or applied via your cosmetics.

Another case in point: all-natural sunscreens with UV protection. Quite a few of these contain zinc oxide and/or oxidized titanium, which are actually minerals that help block the damaging rays from reaching your skin. And while natural minerals may sound blissfully healthy, they're actually quite potent and powerful. (I'm not kidding—for example, you can find oxidized titanium in house paint.) But UV damage is far worse than leaving sunscreen on your skin, so it's preferable to apply sunscreen. Just remember to cleanse it off thoroughly when you're back indoors.

If you're using all natural cosmetics which have no synthetic preservatives, make sure the ingredients don't spoil. Follow the company's directions, such as storing the product in the 'fridge.

Am I saying avoid all-natural products? No. But as a consumer, you should know what you're buying...and what you're putting on your face.

9. SKIN FAST ONCE A WEEK

You've heard of celebrities who go on juice fasts and detox diets in order to flush out their systems and lose pounds quickly, right? Turns out, your skin needs the same break. Remember your skin's natural barrier that protects your skin from dryness, UV rays, pollution, and even cold, biting temperatures? According to Dr. Katayama, advising dermatologist at Mirai Clinical, "Your skin has an inherent ability to take care of itself. If you use moisturizers excessively every day, it causes your skin to become lazy and results in the production of fewer natural oils".

A once-a-week "skin fast" can help your system reboot and keep its natural hydration system in check. (But no more than once a week, please, or you'll risk drying out your skin.) Here, the simple how-to's....

1. Once a week, wash your face gently at night with a mild cleanser.
2. Skip any moisturizers or nighttime wrinkle products and go to sleep "naked". (Yes, pajamas are fine...I'm talking naked skin here!) Optimally, keep your bedroom properly humidified to avoid parching your unprotected skin.
3. In the morning, wash your face gently again, this time using only a splash of lukewarm water. (Note: Try skin fasting on the rest of your skin as well.)
4. Drink plenty of water to compensate for the lack of moisturizing products of the night before.
5. Here's how to test your skin health: Try the morning Tissue Test to determine your true skin type. Simply place a clean tissue over your face; if it sticks, and only begins to fall off as you lean forward, then you have normal skin, which is optimal. However, if it immediately falls off (no

oils to adhere the tissue to your skin), you have a dry complexion. If the tissue is still glued to your face when you're practically looking at the ground, you've got oily skin. In these cases, let's move on to Chapter 10.

10. LESS MOISTURIZER ON DRY SKIN, MORE ON OILY

So far you are doing a great job of protecting your skin's natural moisture barrier by avoiding skin-unfriendly ingredients. You still do need to use moisturizers to replenish the production of natural oils that decrease with age. But how much moisturizer should you use? Here is the answer, now that you've taken the Tissue Test from the previous chapter.

Moisturize oily skin...but leave dry skin alone.

It sounds utterly counterintuitive, but let me explain. There's a difference between "dry" and "dehydrated", and the two words shouldn't be used interchangeably when you're talking about skin.

Dry skin simply means the surface of your skin is thirsty, while underneath it all, your skin might actually be relatively well-hydrated and happily cruising along. That's why it's important to fight the impulse to over-moisturize, which will stifle the production of natural oils and leave you more parched in the long run. Dry skin is made even worse by over-cleansing, which "strips away the natural lipids that account for your skin's moisture," explains Dr. Katayama. So if you fall into that tissue-drops-off-immediately category, scale back the creams and cleansers and let your skin return itself to normal.

Dehydration, on the other hand, means you're parched from the inside (not good) and the tell-tale sign of this condition is what most people refer to as "oily skin". (I know you're probably scratching your head about now.) But logically, it makes sense: underneath the surface, your skin is thirsty, causing the outer layers to desperately protect what little moisture is left by producing excess natural oils. On your end, it's a condition known simply as oily skin, and chances are, you're out buying oil-free makeup and matte powder to compensate for that unsightly sheen. But by significantly increasing your water intake, and using moisturizers diligently, you'll actually rehydrate your skin on an internal level, and are bound to see a reduction in all that excess surface oil.

And, in both cases, continue to Skin Fast once a week.

NO-COST WAYS
TO LOOKING YOUNGER

11. EIGHT AREAS TO WASH WITH SOAP EVERY DAY

There's nothing wrong with wanting your skin to have that fresh-scrubbed, soapy scent that signals clean. But you can have too much of a good thing—even if we're talking about hygiene! When we discussed skin fasting earlier, I explained that overzealous product use could throw off skin's natural balance, causing dryness and/or excess oil production. That's especially true in the cleansing department; all that rubbing, scrubbing, exfoliating, sudsing, and rinsing can strip your complexion of its natural protection barrier, as well as its ability to hold in moisture. Think of it this way: you are literally washing away the best skincare cream in the world, as well as the seal that keeps it in place. Once skin loses that barrier and becomes vulnerable to the elements, you're risking additional environmental damage from UV rays, dry weather, pore-clogging dirt, and damage from harsh, synthetic cosmetic ingredients.

Don't worry, though—I'm not recommending that you skip bathing from here on out. But I am suggesting a specific washing routine that protects every vulnerable area of your body. Here's the rub....

Wash these eight areas each day with a skin-friendly soap (see Chapter 11), as they produce sweat and natural oils which, when oxidized, emit unpleasant odors.

1) the back of your ears
2) behind the neck
3) upper back
4) the décolletage and chest area
5) arm pits
6) groin area and anus
7) feet
8) face

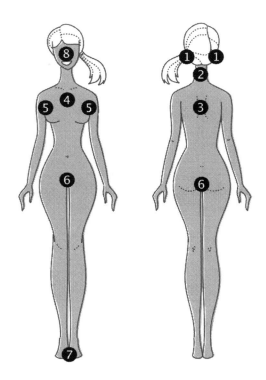

Meanwhile, there's no need to soap up your legs, arms, and stomach—it's perfectly fine to rinse those areas with just water. (Sweat is water-soluble and will rinse right off, while your natural, protective oils stay put.)

Worried you might not have that squeaky-clean smell that everyone loves? Fear not: good bacteria actually prevents the growth of bad (odor-producing) bacteria, so a simple rinse-off shower, sans soap, actually cleanses away less of the good stuff than a sudsy wash. To dry off, pat your body gently with a towel (for your face, use a tissue which is cleaner and gentler). Avoid rubbing, as excessive friction can actually result in an unnaturally darker skin color, like your panty line.

By following this regimen, along with other best skincare practices, you should notice softer and healthier skin within a month.

12. HOW TO GET GROWTH HORMONES, FREE

Read the tabloids and you're likely to hear about the great lengths celebrities go to in order to maintain a young appearance. This often includes injections of synthetic growth hormones (GH), which promote cell rejuvenation when the body's own cell system begins to slow down and help reverse the course of aging by building more lean muscle mass and decreasing body fat.

I'm all for doing everything you can to maintain a youthful appearance, but frankly, synthetic hormones are expensive, controversial, and, as it turns out, unnecessary, since you can actually get a dose of natural GH through exercise. Restocking your own GH levels requires doing activities that produce short, intense, almost explosive bursts of muscle use—think super sets (high repetitions) of weight lifting; lightning-fast sprints up a set of stairs, followed by a walk back down; cranked-up (7.0 mph and higher) speeds on the treadmill for 60 seconds, followed by a one-to-two-minute cool down before you repeat. In fact, studies show that the more muscles you utilize in a single exercise, the more GH you build. Ok, this means a little more work on your part, but think of all the money you can save.

Japanese fitness experts often rely on a unique method of training, called Kaatsu, designed to instantly ramp up GH levels to 290 times more than when you remain still*. Essentially, special belts are attached to specific muscle groups, restricting partial blood flow while you perform a low-intensity movement, such as a tricep curl. (Think about the feeling of a blood-pressure cuff on your arm while you lift a hand weight.) Kaatsu pros claim you can maintain these high levels of GH as long as you practice the method at least once a week. If you have a chance to go to Japan, give it a try.

13. DON'T WASTE ELASTICITY ON A BORING GUY

Remember the old adage, "An ounce of prevention is worth a pound of cure"? When it comes to fighting wrinkles, our grandmothers may have known a thing or two. To understand the concept, I want you to picture two rubber bands: one is brand-spanking new, just out of the box, and has so much spring in it that you could shoot it clear to the next room; the other one has been marinating in a desk drawer for ten years. In fact, when you remove it from the stack of business cards it's been wrapped around, the rubber band—dry and cracked—breaks in your hand. No spring. No elasticity.

The same applies for your skin. Elasticity—the result of elastin protein fibers in the dermis layer—is designed to stretch and shrink back, giving your skin and organs the ability to retain their shape. But just like a rubber band, that elasticity diminishes with time and overuse. Stretch the band again and again, and it becomes lax. Scrunch your face too much and it, too, becomes lax and wrinkled. What am I getting at? It's simple: learn to use your face wisely, preventing those unsightly wrinkles before they take hold. Granted, it won't be easy at first, as you'll have to become conscious of the movements you make, limiting the unnecessary scrunching, pursing, rubbing, and tugging that ultimately leads to—for lack of a better phrase—that "pruney" look. And you'll also need to have some patience, as experts say it can take up to two months to make any new routine a habit. Here, are the easy ground rules....

Feeling confused? Don't let that perplexed state show on your face, in the form of those vertical creases that appear between your eyebrows. Eventually, they'll remain there...even when you're not confused.

- **Looking up from your desk, dinner plate, or book?** Look up with your entire face, not just with your eyes; this prevents the tell-tale forehead creases that form when you lift your eyes only.

- **"Smile smart!"** Just as supermodels learn how to position their lips for the best possible photograph, you can learn to grin in a way that doesn't compromise your skin. Try, for example, smiling without showing your teeth (it's actually an elegant look—especially in pictures); if you do show teeth, go for the uppers only, as revealing all your pearly whites creates smile lines that will require you to invest in injectables down the road.

- **Laugh—but not ear to ear.** The best times in life are those moments when you howl with laughter; just remember to bring your lower jaw down and open wide during those joyous moments, rather than stretching your smile from side to side.

- **Don't waste elasticity on boring guys.** Keeping a smile all the time is great for a positive attitude, but there are times in life when smiling isn't necessary.

Sure, it's a bit of a homework assignment, but the results are well worth it. (And please, no brow-furrowing while you contemplate the task at hand.)

14. A WRINKLE-FREE FACE

What's more effective in reducing wrinkles than any cosmetic product? Training your facial muscles!

Nature has blessed us with an extraordinary set of 33 facial muscles to enable a plethora of facial expressions. Yet, in modern times, we use only 30% of these muscles. When we rely on those same facial muscles over and over again, they tighten and result in wrinkles like the lines between eyebrows, crow's feet, and smile lines.

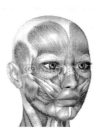

Here are some easy exercises to keep the remaining 70% of your facial muscles in tip-top shape and help keep you looking younger: As in any fitness training, start with the basics, and then keep adding more routines to your repertoire.

Daily Routine #1

Let's first focus on three major areas that show age. This exercise can be incorporated into your evening moisturizing rituals.

Combat Sagging Bulldog Cheeks

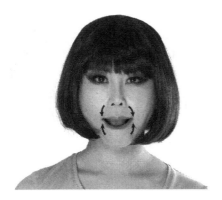

1. Wrap both upper and lower lips around the edges of your teeth to stretch smile lines.

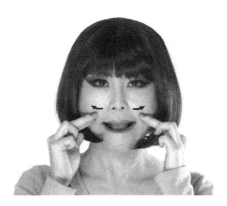

2. Widen your mouth more to pull both sides. Pull up the edges of your mouth.

3. Quickly relax.

4. Do a total of 5 reps Wrap both upper and lower lips around the edges of your teeth to stretch smile lines.

Combat Puffy, Saggy Eyes

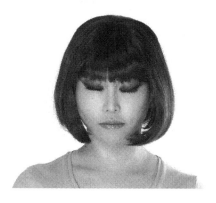

1. Close your eyes firmly without crinkling wrinkles for 5 seconds.

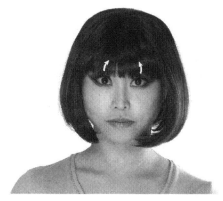

2. Open eyes wide for 5 seconds.

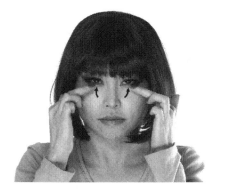

3. Partially close eyes and look up. Tighten your lower eyelid muscle for 5 seconds.

Combat A Turkey Neck

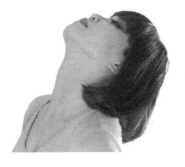

1. Look up.

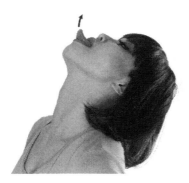

2. Stretch your neck as much as possible and say, "Wooooooooo," for 5 seconds.

Daily Routine #2

Now, let's focus on your lips.

There are two types of muscle: "Fast" muscles are used for instant facial expressions. "Slow" muscles, are used for continuous, extended muscle contractions, and keep your face elastic. Training those slow muscles through lip training is effective for reducing wrinkles and sagging skin.

Facial muscles are generally weak, and since they are not connected to joints, it would be impossible to train each of those 33 facial muscles individually. Because your lip muscles are connected to many other face and neck muscles, training the muscles around your lips activates your other facial muscles, and this exercise will lift up your cheeks and keep your face looking firmer and younger.

It's easy to do lip muscle training while doing any daily activity:

Hold an item in your mouth. Think: pacifier. I hold a bottle cap in my mouth while taking a bath, driving, and even while writing this book! The size of the item you use depends on the size of your mouth. In general, a 1.5-inch diameter object is a good start. This exercise is also good for training nose breathing.

Just be sure not to crinkle your mouth (which forms wrinkles) while holding the item in your mouth. You don't want your skin to "remember" wrinkles. Also, don't use your teeth; just use your lip muscles.

For those of you with x-rated minds, yes, oral sex is great exercise for your lip muscles. Just make sure your partner reciprocates the pleasure!

Daily Routine #3

The Anti-Wrinkle Tongue Trick

Use your tongue to iron out wrinkles and reduce smile lines.

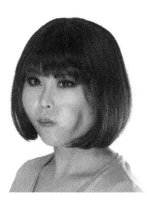

1. Make 10 small circles inside the right side of your mouth with your tongue.

1. Make 10 small circles in the reverse direction.

2. Repeat on the other side of your mouth.

That's it! By doing this, your smile lines are pushed out from the inside. Practicing this exercise after eating or after long periods of speaking (or even laughing a lot) can prevent those smile lines from becoming deeper.

YAWN...

Yawning is the perfect opportunity to train your lip muscles and smile line muscles. So don't waste the chance to train those muscles when you feel that yawn coming on! The trick is to keep your mouth *closed* while yawning.

Use that Toothbrush

Here is a quirky, but effective, way to train lip muscles and reduce smile lines.

After brushing your teeth:

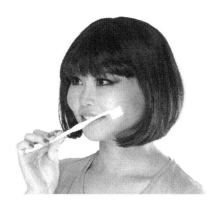

1. Place the toothbrush in your mouth, with the brush facing down.

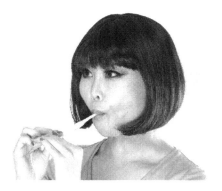

2. Close your mouth, and hold the toothbrush for 10 seconds while attempting to pull it out.

3. Release, and repeat 3 times.

Iron smile lines from the inside out

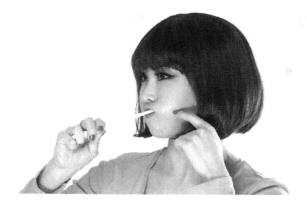

1. Press the back of toothbrush (smooth side) against the inside cheeks of your mouth.

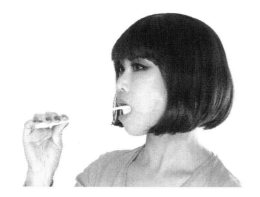

2. Gently massage the inside of your cheeks with the smooth side of the toothbrush in an upward motion.

3. Repeat several times.

4. Repeat on the other side of your mouth.

These simple exercises will help reduce those smile lines. Make your face training a daily habit, and continue these exercises on a regular basis.

15. WRINKLE-FREE HANDS

You can maintain an amazingly young-looking face with skin friendly products, careful daily hygiene, and plenty of sunscreen, but take one glance downward and your hands could be a dead giveaway of your age—literally. Want to keep them youthful looking? A few tips....

A.M. protection: Make it a morning routine and rub cream onto your hands when you moisturize your face. Be sure to bend your fingers so the cream gets into joint crevices.

UV Aging protection: It may seem counterintuitive to put sunscreen on the back of your hands when you're not at the beach, but just think about how much exposure your hands get on a daily basis.

Moisturize whenever hands get wet: In these hygiene-conscious times, frequent hand washing is commonplace. Always follow with a hand cream and be sure to bend your fingers so the cream gets into joint crevices.

Wear gloves whenever possible: Covering your hands is the best possible way to protect them from sun damage, dryness, and harsh cleansing chemicals that can cause wrinkling.

- **When driving:** Slipping on a pair of lightweight cotton gloves is particularly helpful when you're at the wheel; UVA rays penetrate windshield glass and your hands on the steering wheel are prime targets. (Even better, consider investing in a UV-protected windshield filter.)

- **When washing dishes:** Apply moisturizer before you slip on your rubber gloves and you'll literally have a spa going in your kitchen sink. The gloves lock in heat from the hot, sudsy water, creating warmth that allows hand skin to absorb the product you've applied.

- **When sleeping:** Apply a moisturizer and wear lightweight gloves to bed and you'll have (hopefully!) eight full hours for the moisturizer to do its softening magic on your hands.

- **When shampooing your hair:** Ever wonder why stylists wear rubber gloves when you're at the shampoo bowl? They know the importance of protecting hands from the harsh, synthetic cleansing ingredients in shampoo that are designed to rinse away oils. So, why not you? Regular shampoo is not as harmful as the hair color liquid stylists use, but using shampoo almost everyday, will certainly affect your hands.

16. WRINKLE-FREE KNEES

Okay, we know how to keep our face and body looking younger, but let's not forget those two spots which often show the most signs of aging: our elbows and our knees. They tend to get neglected because we can't readily see them, but sagging skin around elbows and knees is a dead giveaway of your age. Even the Japanese jokingly refer to wrinkly elbows and knees as pruney Japanese plums!

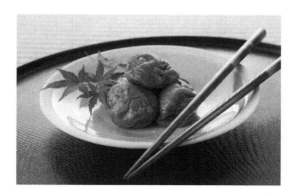

To reduce wrinkles on your knees (which, like those on your face, are the result of UV exposure, poor muscle tone, and low metabolism), scrub them to get rid of dead cells, and follow with a skin-friendly moisturizer.

While muscle training doesn't do much for reducing wrinkly elbows, it is effective in preventing sagging of the skin above the knees.

Here are two easy, anti-wrinkly knee exercises to do while sitting at your desk.

Exercise #1

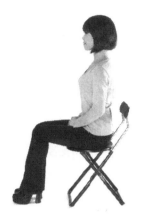

1. Sit with a straight back and hold the chair with both hands to stabilize your body.

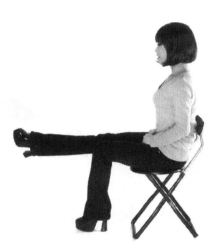

2. (See photo left): Raise one straight leg to knee level, while keeping your toes bent, and hold for 10 seconds.

3. Repeat with the other leg.

4. Do a total of 5 sets.

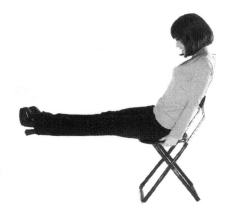

5. If you can, raise the both legs and hold for 10 seconds.

Exercise #2

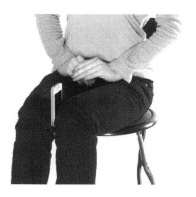

While sitting, hold an object such as the phone or a piece of paper between your knees as long as possible to train your inner thigh muscles.

17. A WRINKLE-FREE NECK

Nothing looks more awkward than a wrinkle-free face atop a crepey neck that's been neglected. Believe it or not, your pillow may be the biggest culprit, causing sleep lines to form and deepen at night, eventually etching them permanently into your skin. Follow these pillow tips and you'll reduce the wrinkling significantly:

Avoid sleeping on a high pillow. You may love the feel or support, but it forces an angle that creates lines in your neck skin.

- **Readjust your reading posture in bed.** Instead of propping yourself up against pillows (which brings your chin down), consider lying almost flat and putting a pillow on your chest to prop your book into an upright position so it's at eye level.

- **Consider a buckwheat pillow.** Buckwheat is good in noodles, and even better in pillows! The Japanese love buckwheat in bed for a number of reasons: it's a natural, inexpensive, and renewable resource; it provides excellent head, neck, and back support; and it allows for air circulation that results in a peaceful night's rest. You can find them online from a number of reputable websites.

- **Be mindful about keeping your chin upright all day long.** Whether you're walking, working on a computer, or texting on your phone, make an effort to gaze straight ahead.

18. A WRINKLE-FREE VOICE

Ever notice how an elderly person's voice often has a halting, quavering quality to it? It's a natural progression for the vocal cords, which atrophy and weaken with age, causing that familiar hoarseness that makes us sound, well, old. Fortunately, you can apply anti-aging strategies to your voice—just like you would your face or body—and turn back the hands of time in the vocal department. Doing so might even have interpersonal benefits, according to psychologist Albert Mehrabian, whose studies found that 38 percent of perception is based purely on verbal impression.

- **Breathe from your diaphragm:** It's a technique that's routinely used by singers--who rely 70 percent on their abdominal muscles and only 30 percent on their vocal cords--to produce a deep, clear resonance. By expanding your abdomen and reaching deep down for sound, you'll have an easier time controlling the volume of your voice and avoid inflamed vocal cords, which result in hoarseness. (You naturally do this when you lie down on your back, as your abdomen expands and your shoulders stay flat.)

- **Work your abs:** When you train your core and abdominal muscles, you'll have an easier time producing that desirable depth of sound. (Not sure how you sound? Record your voice on your phone and give a listen.) Just breathing from your diaphragm helps build ab muscles as it uses transverse ab muscles, called a "natural corset", that cover your abs. Since people breath 20,000 times per day, you will be training your abs 20,000 times per day!

- **Keep quiet in the mornings:** Vocal cords are dry for the first three hours after you awaken, so give them a rest (until they warm up) to avoid excess strain and inflammation.

- **Steer clear of overly-dry environments:** When you speak, your vocal cords literally vibrate; and if they're parched, that vibration can cause damage. (Think of a brittle branch banging against a tree trunk.) If your home is dry, consider placing a humidifier in your room at night.

- **Try neck exercises:** Your vocal cords are surrounded by throat muscles; give them a workout. Try my "anti-turkey neck" maneuver in Chapter 17, and you'll strengthen your cords at the same time.

- **Go smoke-free:** We all know the cancer-causing effects of cigarettes, but those butts wreak havoc on your vocal cords, too, sapping them of the moisture and suppleness that produce a resonant sound. (Seriously— I've heard some smokers go as far as having hyaluronic acid injected into their cords to replace the moisture the cigarettes draw out. Easier to just quit smoking?)

EAT YOUR WAY TO WEIGHT LOSS

19. PORTION CONTROL, THE JAPANESE WAY

We all know that the Japanese have a different daily diet than most Americans—while you're downing a morning bowl of Special K, I'm happily downing a bowl of rice and tofu. But how we eat is different, too, and it's a key component in our ability to maintain a healthy body weight. The good news is that no matter what kinds of foods you're consuming on a daily basis, it's easy to adapt to the Japanese way of eating and begin to bring balance and portion control into your life. Here are some smart rules that I try to follow each and every day:

- **Replace the dinner plate with many small-size dishes:** You wouldn't think that a simple plate gets in the way of healthy eating, but, in fact, it lacks the cues for balance and portion control that the Japanese rely on to control their weight. Here's why: we derive a lot of satisfaction from food served in a way that's pleasing to the eye—it slows down our eating, makes us fully aware of what we're putting in our mouths, and provides a focus other than quickly scarfing down the food. By composing a meal with lots of little bowls and mini plates, we're building the meal from a visual standpoint...and avoiding relying on a giant dinner plate that gets smothered with oversize portions.

- **Create meals with a variety of flavors, textures, and colors:** Think about how many times you've gorged yourself on a heaping bowl of mac-n-cheese or spaghetti. I'm betting that halfway through the meal, all that pasta lost the delicious impact of the first few bites, yet you probably continued to eat until you saw the bottom of the bowl. That doesn't happen in Japan very often, because we literally tantalize our palate with constant surprises: a citrusy mound of pickled cucumbers...a tidbit of savory fish...a soothing scoop of rice. While it appears to be a profusion of food on the table, in reality, we're eating fewer calories than the average American meal. So, when eating out, order several small appetizers rather than a large main course.

- **Eat until you're 80-percent full—then stop!** From early childhood on, most Americans hear admonishments about the starving children in (fill-in-the-country), and are encouraged to "eat up" and "clean your plate". Problem is, doing so only serves to over-feed you (and, might I add, does nothing to help improve the lives of the impoverished, and obesity adds pressures on the government's healthcare budget). The Japanese, on the other hand, are taught to move mindfully from dish to dish, strategically pacing themselves so they are in tune with the feeling of satiety that kicks in before you finish your entire meal. (Eat too fast and you will have gobbled everything up before your stomach has signaled to your brain that you're full.)

- **Use small-size flatware or even chopsticks:** Face it, the less food you can fit on your fork or spoon, the slower you'll eat. Chopsticks automatically force you to reduce the size of your bites; and for those who aren't accustomed to eating with them, chopsticks offer that unhurried pace that keeps you in tune with your "full meter". Be sure, too, to put down your utensils between bites, savoring each bit of food in your mouth, and chewing thoroughly before moving on to the next bite.

- **Work up to 30 chews:** It might sound laborious at first, but start with ten chews and work your way up. Not only does this chew-fest slow down your pace and satisfy your appetite more quickly, but the increased saliva will activate digestive enzymes (which lead to satiety); release a growth hormone, known as Parotin, that rejuvenates muscles, bone, and teeth; and give your mouth muscles a good workout that helps to ward off facial sag down the road. If that doesn't make the case for a few extra chomps on your sandwich today, I don't know what will.

- **Have a mini dessert:** By now, you've probably seen the proliferation of Japanese buffet restaurants in America, which always showcase a tantalizing dessert section, filled to the brim with tiny, one-inch by one-inch tidbits of cheesecake, tiramisu, and chocolate fudge cake. Those Lilliputian treats aren't a budget decision...they're actually the Japanese style of serving dessert in minimalist portions that limit gorging on sweets. Follow the habit of a small taste after dinner, and you'll keep your taste buds happy while shaving off hundreds of calories in the process. Don't just eat it, taste it!

20. EAT YOUR VEGGIES FIRST!
YOUR EATING ORDER MATTERS

Your mom wasn't kidding when she urged you to eat your vegetables...but what she might not have known is that it's important to eat them before you go on to the rest of your meal. (And I'm not just talking about the dinner salad before your entrée.) There's serious science behind this advice—which may explain all the diet books that talk about eating foods in specific combinations--but I'll try to simplify things here so you're not tempted to skip to the next chapter!

You've probably heard that simple carbohydrates (i.e., "starches", like white bread, white pasta, and white rice) convert to sugars when we eat them, sending a surge of insulin directly into your bloodstream. That's great for a runner about to embark on an energetic sprint...but it's not so great for your skin, because "those sugar molecules cling to protein molecules, and in doing so, break down the vital collagen fibers that are the backbone of a youthful complexion", says Charlene Brannon, Ph.D., scientific advisor to Mirai Clinical. (Need a visual? Think of the collagen fibers in your face as a tightly knit tarp...but as time goes on, the holes in the tarp get bigger and looser. Anything that weakens those fibers will show up as loose skin and wrinkles on your face.) This collagen-breaking process is known as Glycation...and you want to avoid it at all costs.

Which leads us back to the veggies: if your stomach is busy digesting that first course of fiber-rich vegetables, any carb that comes down the pike will literally be covered with those fibers, inhibiting their ability to cling to the proteins and therefore wreak havoc on your skin. There's a weight-loss bonus here as well, because the fiber minimizes insulin spikes (which store fat), and will help you feel fuller.

The Japanese "Kaiseki", is a traditional, multi-course meal that always starts with vegetables. You can adapt this approach to your diet fairly easily. When the waiter places the white bread basket on your table before you've had anything else to eat, consider asking him to remove it and wait for fresh greens or a tomato salad to begin your meal instead; then go on to enjoy the rest of your meal. Your waistline, and your face, will thank you for it.

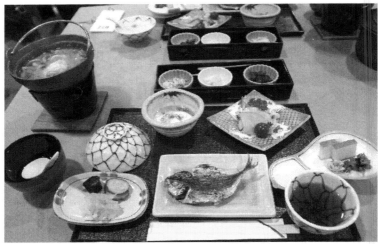

Traditional Japanese Kaiseki

21. THE 30-FOODS-PER-DAY RULE

In Chapter 19, we talked about creating variety in your daily meals. The Japanese take that a bit further. We are taught to eat 30 foods per day—small in quantity, but large in variety—a strategy that maximizes the absorption of nutrition, and helps keep you feeling full longer.

Let's take a look at an average daily diet in Japan vs. a typical American meal plan:

The Japanese breakfast:

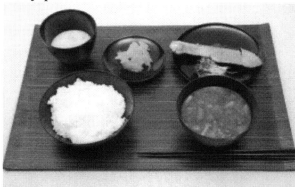

- Daikon radish
- Eggs with soy sauce
- Salmon and sprouts
- Rice
- Miso soup with mushrooms

The Japanese lunch:

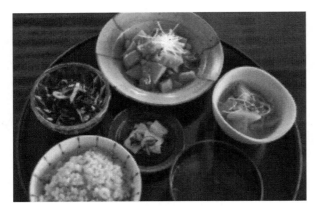

- Hijiki salad with seaweed, carrots, cucumber, sesame, sugar, rice wine, and soy sauce
- Mixed vegetable dish with lotus root, daikon, green pepper, carrots, beans, and shiitake mushrooms
- Salad of daikon and sprouts, with sake, mirin (rice wine), and soy sauce dressing
- Brown rice
- Daikon with spinach and turnips

The Japanese dinner:

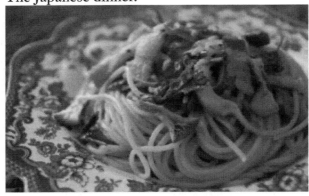

- Pasta dish with mushrooms and bacon

- Soy, basil, olive oil, and garlic

The American breakfast:

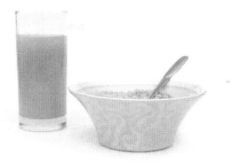

- Cereal with milk
- Glass of orange juice

The American lunch:

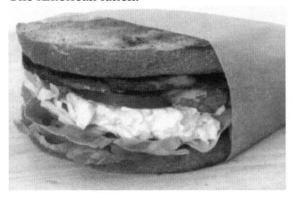

- Egg-salad sandwich with bacon, lettuce, and tomato on toasted whole wheat bread

The American dinner:

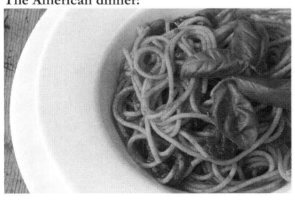

- Spaghetti with marinara sauce and a basil garnish

Were you counting? You can see the differences right away. The Japanese meals included 26 different foods, while the American meal plan featured only 11. Examine the components of the meals closely and you'll also notice that the Japanese version managed to include 17 different vegetables, while the American diet had just three.

"The key is small portions of each but more variety. Nutrients always work better in a team. They don't work well individually. The more nutrients you get, the more absorption you get from the nutrients," says Dr. Charlene Brannon, former professor of food chemistry at the University of Washington and Mirai Clinical's scientific advisor.

And chances are, with all those fiber-rich veggies...satisfying, low-calorie options like soup...and the visual appeal of variety, the Japanese breakfast would keep you going for five hours, whereas the stateside option would leave you feeling hungry long before the lunch bell rings.

It's easy to adjust your own meals to reflect this healthy, weight-conscious way of eating. You might, for example, throw a handful of blueberries on your morning cereal; add a side salad to your lunch sandwich; and round out your dinner pasta with a topping of chicken and a side of broccoli. But remember to reduce the quantity of the other existing foods, such as the pasta, so your total calorie intake is not excessive. The changes are easy... but significant.

22. THE BENEFIT OF "THE BENTO BOX" LUNCH

One of the easiest ways the Japanese remind themselves to eat within the 30-food-per-day rule is to serve their meals in what's known as a Bento Box----essentially a multi-compartmentalized food tray designed to showcase an entrée dish alongside a variety of accompaniments. It's a truly visual way to make certain that your lunch meal consists of a large assortment of proteins, vegetables, and carbohydrates.

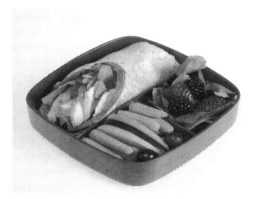

That said, the Bento has a whole host of other attributes that lead to good health, weight loss, a happy pocketbook, and even well-fed kids. Here's why the box is tops...

It forces you to find balance: Fill up your plate at a traditional American meal, and you might well be tempted to take a huge portion of that meaty pot roast, a pile of mashed potatoes, and then fill the tiny space that remains with a few measly leaves of salad. Serve your meal in a Bento, on the other hand, and you'll be guided to automatically re-portion the foods you prepare. The main compartment, for example, won't hold as much meat, fish, or other protein as you might be tempted to put on your plate; the side sections are equally discriminating.

- **You know what you're eating:** In this day of preservatives, unhealthy fast food, and a "hefty" reliance on restaurant meals, it's gratifying to pack your own healthy, colorful lunch and feel good about the fact that there are no hidden surprises in the food you put into your body.

- **You'll get portion control:** Because the amounts are pre-set when you fill the box, there's no temptation to overeat, serve yourself seconds, or over-order a multi-course meal.

- **The Bento is budget-friendly:** It's the perfect way to capitalize on leftovers (that piece of salmon, say), and pump up your meal with some additional veggies—no restaurant bill in sight.

- **It saves precious time:** No more running out and standing on line for takeout food at lunch, nor waiting for a restaurant meal to be served. The Bento is a neat, tidy, healthy way to eat a wide variety of foods right at your desk.

- **Kids love the lively presentation:** Good nutrition starts at a young age, and if you put a slice of pizza, chicken nuggets, or a fatty hot dog in front of a child, chances are, they'll gobble it up. But pack an adorable Character-Bento or Chara-Ben (the Japanese term to describe food characters that moms often prepare for their children), and your kids are likely to be just as enthusiastic about the lunch in front of them. Simply find a playful Bento Box (they're often inscribed with characters like Pokemon or Hello Kitty), and trick out the foods with fun faces, such as a tomato nose and carrot ears on a scoop of rice. Now *that's* my idea of a Happy Meal!

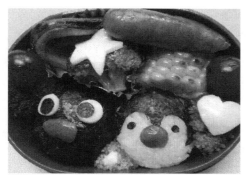

Children's Bento Box

23. THE NINJA BLACK DIET

I know...most people think of Ninjas as those uber-cool movie superheroes in skin-tight black suits. But the fact of the matter is, Ninjas were actually 15th-century Japanese warriors, trained in unorthodox arts of war. They were superbly strong, flexible, and fast—able to beat the enemy at a moment's notice. And there was a reason for their power and strength (which didn't come from a costume, by the way!): Ninjas, like many Japanese today, ate according to color; meaning, they chose darker foods (also known as "warm" foods) over white ("cold") foods.

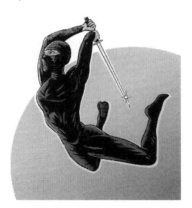

First of all, it's important to know that I'm not talking about the foods being physically warm or cold (whether you heat them up or not is irrelevant here). The thinking behind nutritional color theory is that darker foods improve blood circulation, increase metabolism, and enhance your general health.

They range from black to brown to deep, rich tones of orange, purple, red, and green. Some examples:

- Black or brown rice, quinoa, and barley
- Whole-wheat or multi-grain bread
- Whole-wheat pasta
- Brown sugar and agave nectar
- Black beans and black sesame seeds
- Dark malt vinegar
- Dark beer
- Vegetables: pumpkin, carrots, and other root vegetables
- Fruits: cherries, blueberries, strawberries and plums
- Fish and seafood: shrimp, mackerel, salmon, sardines, tuna, herring, and yellowtail
- Meat: lamb, chicken, egg, beef, ham, bacon, sausage, and pork

Stay with me here. These "warm", black or darker-colored foods, tend to be grown in colder climates and are thought to have properties which warm the body, while "cold", white or lighter colored foods, tend to be grown in (you got it!) warmer climates and are thought to cool down the body.

While it's important to eat a balance of warm and cold foods (in fact, some of the Japanese superfoods mentioned in the "Your Dietary BFF's" section are considered cold), I find that most people actually have a warm deficiency...often due to lack of exercise, poor diet, exposure to air conditioning, and even genetics. (This can manifest itself as low blood pressure, a sluggish metabolism, excess fat, water retention, and digestive troubles like diarrhea or constipation.) So next time you head to the kitchen, or sit down with a restaurant menu, try to incorporate as many potent "warm" – the darker colored—foods into your diet as possible... you'll be helping to keep your body in tip-top shape, with renewed energy, and glowing skin. Turns out those Ninjas knew a thing or two about staying "in fighting shape".

24. LOSE WEIGHT BY STAYING WARM

I'm sure you know that increased metabolism burns more calories. But did you know that just by increasing your body temperature by 1C/1.8F, you could increase your body's metabolism by 12%?

So, it makes sense to keep your body temperature on the warm side even when you're not exercising or in the gym. Ideally, your body should register between 33.2 – 38.2 C/92-101 F. (Drop below 35 C/95 F, and you actually decrease your resistance to infection by 40 percent, and increase your risk of contracting diseases like cancer.) Warm yourself up a bit (by just 1 C/1.8 F), and the benefits are plentiful: your basal metabolic rate (BMR), which is your metabolism when you're at rest, increases by 12 percent, and your immune system cranks up by a whopping 60 percent. Turns out, it's cool to not be cool!

Here, some tips to warm up your system...

- **Avoid air conditioning:** That chilly blast may feel good, but it's not doing you any favors in the health and fitness department. So when the sun comes out, resist the urge to cool down your home, car, and office, or at the very least, keep the temperature at a moderate level.

- **Exercise regularly:** Not only will you be revving up your metabolism and burning calories, but you'll build muscles and a healthy heart at the same time.

- **Avoid cold drinks:** Quaffing too many icy beverages cools you down from the inside out.

- **Limit white sugar and simple carbohydrates:** According to Eastern medicine, these high-glycemic foods are said to reduce your body temperature—which is yet another reason to swap unhealthy choices like white bread for the complex carbs of whole grain.

- **Stick to baths:** A nice, warm soak in the tub elevates your body temperature faster and more effectively than a quick hop in the shower.

- **Steer clear of tight underwear:** In old-school Japan, men used to actually don a diaper-like garment known as fundoshi in lieu of traditional underwear, which helped avoid cutting off blood circulation. These days, the trend has taken hold amongst Japanese women, who like the comfort of this non-traditional "pant".

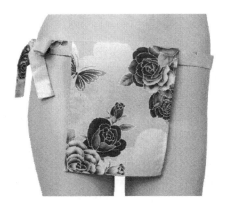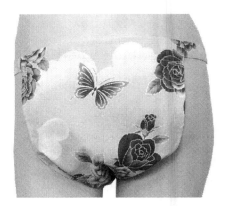

Loose underwear supports healthy blood circulation

25. FAT-BURNING WHILE BATHING

Temperature and weight loss are intricately connected. Despite the fact that warmer body temperatures are equated with good health, many Japanese have actually learned to manipulate their fat cells (brown) and fat-storing cells (white) for maximum efficiency by following a warm bath with a cold bath plunge, followed by a warm soak.

When your body temperature is suddenly reduced for a short time, your brown cells spring into action, burning energy like your own personal furnace in order to create heat within your body. In other words: you're shivering and your body, working hard to bring up the temperature, is peeling off calories in the process. That chilly state also helps rev up circulation, as your body wildly pumps blood through those arteries and veins in an attempt to warm things up. When you feel warm, on the other hand, your body produces Heat Shock Proteins (HSP), a cell-repair mechanism—with anti-aging benefits such as producing collagen for skin--that kick in when your cells are exposed to elevated temperatures. (Want proof? Take a look at the skinny Japanese wild monkeys that roam near volcano and hot spring areas; they routinely expose their bodies to hot water...then jump into the cold snow immediately afterwards. It's like their very own weight-management program!)

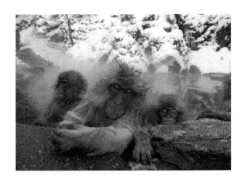

All of this explains why the key to revving up those internal engines lies in alternately increasing and decreasing body temperature. It's a natural habit for the Japanese, given that we've always loved bathing rituals. Even Samurai warriors were said to have soaked in hot mineral springs to heal battle injuries. (We refer to this ritual, by the way, as "yuji"; "yu" means hot water, and "ji" means healing.) To this day, hot springs are in abundance in our country, one of the few upsides to the unstable geological environment that's been responsible for our catastrophic tsunamis and earthquakes.

In Japan, we typically turn to the bath for both physical and mental relaxation, beginning with body washing and rinsing before we enter the pristine tub (known as a "furo") for a luxurious, warm soak. After this, we often begin the hot/cold regimen that jump-starts the metabolism...generally in this order: hot bath, cold shower, hot bath, cold shower. Feel free to alter the routine based on your personal preference: if you want to wake yourself up and get a bit of a jolt, I advise ending with cold; but if it's relaxation you're after (say, you're about to go to bed after a long, hard day), finish up with the hot bath.

YOUR DIETARY BFF'S

26. GOOD SKIN IS THE SIGN OF GOOD HEALTH

The old adage, "Beauty comes from within..." is more than just a saying; it's a physiological fact. That's because it's impossible to have good, clear, glowing skin without being healthy. Need proof? Just take a look at the complexion of someone who is exhausted, stressed, or fighting a virus or infection. Chances are, that person's skin looks pale or sallow; he or she might be experiencing breakouts, have dark circles under the eyes, and lack that glow we all strive for.

The good nutrients found in the food you digest first go towards rejuvenating, conditioning, and healing your internal organs, muscles, and blood. Then the leftover nutrients are delivered to the outside, your skin. So, it stands to reason that if your insides need a lot of work, there won't be much left for your outsides.

On the other hand, if you take care of yourself on a physiological level—through good nutrition, regular exercise, and regular check-ups—your skin will automatically show the results.

27. FOOD AS MEDICINE

Consuming the wrong foods can cause disease, and eating the right foods can cure disease.

Today, modern science and medicine have begun to agree with this ancient wisdom. More and more, people are realizing that diet is directly connected to their health and well-being. There is a greater recognition of how the food we eat, what it is made of and how it is prepared, affects us. This holistic point of view is a very important part of the traditional Japanese way of eating.

Japanese cuisine, though no longer untouched by industrialized food processing techniques, is still one of the healthiest in the world. By stocking up on the Japanese foods that heal, your kitchen pantry will literally become a medicine chest. Many of these foods, such as green tea, miso, shiitake and maitake mushrooms, tofu, and edamame, have been scientifically proven to cure and prevent degenerative disease and to prevent aging. Vegetables from the sea are nature's mineral storehouse. Foods such as seitan (wheat gluten) and tofu are great substitutes for less healthy sources of protein, such as meat and dairy.

The evolution in scientific information about diet and our health and well-being has produced a whole new field of study devoted to what are now called medicinal or "functional" foods – foods that have potential benefits beyond their traditional nutritional value. These foods contain high concentrations of phytochemicals – natural plant substances that have been shown effective in the treatment and prevention of degenerative disease. Many of these phytochemicals are important to the plant's own survival. The powerful immune-boosting biochemicals found in shiitake and maitake mushrooms are nature's way of protecting these fungi from being destroyed by the natural defense mechanisms of their host. (Ironically, as plants have evolved and adapted to survive and meet the challenges of their varied environments, they have become important to our own health and survival.)

You are what you eat. If you want to cure your disease or any disorder, first eat right, instead of relying on a drug. In general, drugs cure the symptoms quickly but not the cause. So, in order to keep your health in good condition, you may have to keep taking the drug forever. That's such a great system for drug companies, but not for you. You should become healthy by eating correctly, therefore curing the cause of the illness by yourself.

"Yakuzen" ("medical food" in Japanese) focuses on the environment in which people live, the climate, the physical environment, and the seasons of the region. The physical constitution of an individual is also considered when creating a meal adapted to these factors, in addition to the special medicinal properties of the ingredients being used.

Yakuzen has a 1000 year history. It is a form of pharmacotherapy that is unique to Japanese and Chinese herbs that aims at both prevention and treatment of disease. Yakuzen was established according to the theory of Chinese medicine based on an accumulation of experience with diets containing Chinese herbal medicines, and profound knowledge of Chinese medicine. Records of medicinal porridge can be traced back to ancient times, and it is even mentioned in a chapter in the first book on medicine in China.

It seems appropriate to regard Yakuzen therapy as diet therapy. Yakuzen comprises a variety of elements, including medicinal porridge, medicinal tea, and medicinal liquor, and it occupies an important position in Japanese and Chinese medicine. Dialectic serving of Yakuzen is an approach that serves Yakuzen taking into account various elements, including the patient's condition, season, and living environment, on the basis of dialectics. Yakuzen has so many rules, but one of the main rules of Yakuzen is to eat "cold" or "warm" foods depending on your health condition, which is explained in Chapter 23.

28. SUSHI IS NOT JUST TASTY

Wherever you travel in the U.S., you are likely to find a sushi bar. I'm always amazed by the how extensive and creative sushi menus have become, but for sushi to remain healthy and effective for weight loss, only the most authentically "nigiri" style Japanese sushi will do: that is, the simplest ones with sushi rice and pieces of raw fish. Please go ahead and enjoy the fancier versions like spider rolls and the ubiquitous California rolls, but keep in mind these are not diet-friendly. Here's what makes nigiri sushi so healthy:

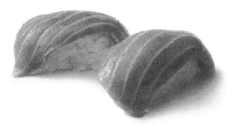

- Fish Oil
  Fish, like salmon and mackerel, is loaded with those beneficial oils—Omega-3 fatty acids (EPA, DHA)—which help support heart and brain health. These fatty acids also help improve skin cell rejuvenation and help to retain moisture in the skin. While you can get these vital nutrients through supplements, nutrition is most efficiently gained from real foods. (Excessive eating of tuna in the U.S. should be avoided due to its potential mercury content.)

- Raw Food Enzymes
  Raw fish is loaded with metabolism-boosting enzymes, which are destroyed when foods are heated.

- Lean Protein
  Raw fish is an excellent source of lean protein, necessary for healthy muscle and skin, and it contains very little heart-clogging saturated fat.

- Ginger
  One of the best foods for healthy digestion and blood circulation, ginger should be eaten before sushi, because sushi often uses white rice, a "cold" food which can lower your body temperature. Eating ginger before sushi also reduces glycation and insulin spikes. (If there is no ginger served with your sushi, have miso soup or seaweed salad before eating sushi.)

- Wasabi (Japanese Horseradish)
  New research shows that allyl isothiocyanate (AITC), a compound abundant in wasabi, helps to reduce the risk of bladder cancer.* Wasabi and ginger both have antibacterial qualities.

- Nori, Seaweed Wrap
  Another popular type of sushi is the "maki" or sushi roll. Nori, the seaweed wrap used, is rich in essential vitamins and minerals.

- Vinegar
  As you have learned in the Ninja Diet (Chaper 23), white rice is not as preferable as brown rice, nor is it as nutritious. But sushi rice is made with rice wine vinegar, which includes citric acid, known to ease fatigue and increase metabolism. Vinegar also minimizes any insulin spike from white rice, so you don't have to worry about eating white rice if vinegar has been used in preparation.

You may have heard stories of women losing weight by eating only sushi, but please keep in mind that effective weight loss, the Japanese way, also includes eating a wide variety of foods in small portions. Whenever you take a bite of delicious sushi, remember all the good healthy nutrients you are receiving!

*Bhattacharya, A, Y Li, KL Wade, JD Paonessa, JW Fahey and Y Zhang. 2010. Allyl isothiocyanate-rich mustard seed powder inhibits bladder cancer growth and muscle invasion.

29. HEALTH & BEAUTY IN A CUP OF GREEN TEA

For centuries, all tea was green tea, the leaves of the camellia sinensis plant. The fascination with green tea was followed much later with oolong, black and other kinds of Asian teas.

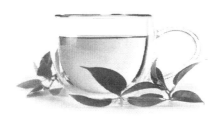

Our forbearers knew the wondrous health benefits of green tea and always drank this natural beverage, not only as an accompaniment to food, but as medicine.

Green tea is bursting with catechins, a group of powerful polyphenols or plant antioxidants that are documented to have amazing health benefits.

Modern Western science has even confirmed the health-giving benefits of our favorite green brew. Green tea helps treat and/or prevent a gamut of diseases such as multiple sclerosis, diabetes, several types of cancer, Alzheimer's disease, Parkinson's disease, heart attacks and heart disease, arthritis, and high blood cholesterol. It strengthens a flagging immunity, and protects your pearly whites by killing the bacteria that causes plaque.

Recent studies show that green tea is effective in slowing down weight gain associated with a high-fat diet. It ramps up your metabolism and dissolves midsection fat.

Sugary drinks, on the other hand, are known to spike blood sugar levels. Too much insulin in the bloodstream leads to diabetes, overweight/obesity, and premature aging. It causes tooth decay, malnutrition, ulcers, kidney problems, and systemic acidosis. Fizzy, carbonated drinks are also notorious for causing osteoporosis because soda increases calcium excretion in the urine which displaces the nutritional value in calcium-rich beverages like milk. Maybe sodas are called 'soft drinks' because they soften the bones! In addition, aspartame or other artificial sweeteners, which are common in soft drinks, are known for their health risks, too.

So, make green tea a staple of your daily diet, and be rewarded with its numerous health benefits including fresh, glowing skin, and a slim waistline.

30. EDAMAME, A MENOPAUSE SUPER FOOD

Japanese women rarely use their word for "menopause" in conversations. This is because they are known to experience less menopausal symptoms than their western counterparts. For example, because of their lack of symptoms such as hot flashes and mood swings, as little as 1.5% of women in Japan* undergo hormone replacement therapy, compared to 40% of women in the U.S.

This lower degree of menopausal symptoms might be largely attributed to the inclusion of soy foods in the Japanese diet. Soy contains phytoestrogens, specifically isoflavones. During perimenopause or menopause, when women's estrogen levels start to fluctuate or decrease, soy's phytoestrogens perform a sort of balancing act by acting like weak estrogens, and help her to maintain a healthful hormonal balance.

Soy's isoflavones may provide just enough estrogenic activity to prevent or reduce uncomfortable symptoms, like hot flashes. In addition, research suggests that soy isoflavones may also promote the reabsorption of bone and therefore inhibit postmenopausal osteoporosis, and that a moderate consumption of soy can help reduce the risk of breast cancer. The FDA even allows certain soy products (with at least 6.25 grams of soy protein per serving) to have a "heart-healthy" claim on their labels.

As protein is the building block of your skin, protein-rich soy benefits skin health. "Estrogen is connected to collagen and elastin production which is essential for healthy skin. It keeps your skin, hair, and nails healthy. That's why during menopause, you might suffer from dry or flaky skin", says Dr. Kato, advising dermatologist for Mirai Clinical.

89

Soybeans, first grown in tropical Asia thousands of years ago, are used in an enormous range of everyday Japanese staples such as soy sauce, vegetable oils, tofu, and miso. The Japanese eat more soy than anyone else in the world. The next chapters will talk about other forms of soy foods, but let me start with my favorite healthy snack.

If you go to a kind of informal Japanese restaurant called "Izakaya" for a drink after work, you are often served edamame, cooked soybeans-in-their-shell, as an appetizer. You might think it's because edamame is so tasty, but there's another reason why alcoholic drinks and edamame are often served together: edamame is known to help purify toxins in the liver.

Besides having edamame with a drink to help protect your liver, make it one of your go-to snacks. Frozen edamame is now found in mainstream grocery stores (try to find the organic ones), and are quick to prepare as appetizers. You can eat them right out of their shells (be sure not to eat the shell itself!) or add the shelled beans to salads.

Soy is most potent when it has been fermented. Fermentation concentrates the power of the healthy plant estrogens found in soy and converts them into a form that our bodies can use more easily, which makes fermented soy even healthier than tofu or soy milk. Common forms of fermented soy are soy sauce and miso.

One type of soy that the Japanese relish (but it really takes getting used to by Westerners) is a Natto, the fermented soybean. Natto is an ugly-looking and stinky food, but it's so highly nutritious and rich in protein that I must mention it. In fact, natto has recently received keen attention because of its natural enzyme, nattokinase. Even American companies have started to market Nattokinase supplements.

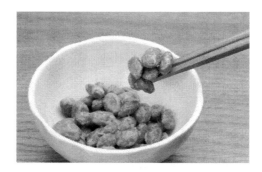

Nattokinase has been shown to reduce the risk of blood clots and help break up the plaque in the brain associated with Alzheimer's disease.

In Japan, people routinely enjoy natto for breakfast, served on top of rice with an egg split over it. You can find it at health food stories, Asian markets, or online.

Try it!

* NPO Women and Menopause, Treatments for menopause among countries, 2009
http://www.meno-sg.net/iryou/kaigai-1.html

31. SEAWEED, THE EDIBLE COSMETIC

We talked about nori in the Sushi chapter, but let me tell you more about other types of seaweed and their remarkable benefits. Overall, the iodine in seaweed improves thyroid function which supports skin rejuvenation, better metabolism, and weight loss.

There are several kinds of seaweed available in supermarkets. One of the most popular ones is "wakame", a major type of seaweed in Japan which is enjoyed for its flavor and health benefits. In Japanese, "WAKA" means "young" and "ME" is "shoot of plants". Indeed, wakame will help keep you young!

Despite being chockful of minerals and nutrients, wakame has almost zero calories. Although high in sodium, it is a good source of other minerals including magnesium, calcium, and iron, and it's high in vitamins A, C, E, and K as well as folate and riboflavin. As it's also a source of lignans, thought to play a role in preventing certain types of cancer, it's not surprising that the Japanese who eat wakame seaweed on a frequent basis have one of the lowest breast cancer rates in the world.

Its high iodine content is especially important for the normal functioning of the thyroid gland. An overactive thyroid typically leads to unhealthy weight loss, nervousness, tremors, heart palpitations, and excessively high body temperatures, whereas an inactive thyroid leads to weight gain, severe fatigue, dry skin, lethargy, and colder hands and feet.

Respective to weight loss, studies show that an ingredient found in wakame known as fucoxanthin promotes weight loss by increasing the rate at which fat is broken down.

Fresh wakame is served in all Japanese restaurants, as an appetizer or in miso soups. Wakame in its dry form can be purchased in packages at most health food stores and natural food markets. It quickly expands, softens, and makes a flavorful addition when added to soups during preparation. See my favorite wakame salad recipe below.

NORI, the dark green flat sheets of seaweed used for sushi, has almost the same benefits as wakame, and is associated with lower rates of breast cancer for both pre-menopausal and menopausal women (as well as lowering blood cholesterol levels).

Here is my skin-rejuvenating wakame salad recipe:

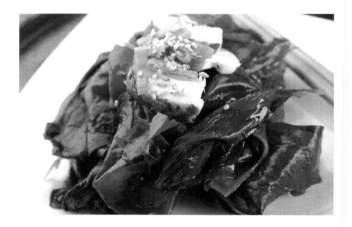

1. Slice a cucumber (the more adventurous can add sliced, cooked, protein-rich octopus).
2. Soak dry wakame and drain as directed on the package.
3. Combine the ingredients.
4. Mix in rice wine vinegar, a pinch of sugar and salt, a soy source, and sesame seeds to taste.

32. SHIITAKE, THE MEDICAL MUSHROOM

Long revered for it's healing and medicinal qualities in Asia, the Shiitake mushroom is making its way into Western lifestyles.

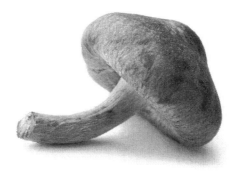

The polysaccharide in shiitake is the source of the mushroom's ability to control blood sugar to help manage diabetes and improve weight loss. In addition, shiitake is full of fiber, which helps prevent constipation and makes you feel full longer.

Shiitake mushrooms play an important role in supporting the immune function. One especially interesting area of support involves the impact of shiitake mushrooms on immune cells called macrophage which are responsible for identifying and clearing potentially cancerous cells from the body, especially those related to prostate cancer, breast cancer, and colon cancer.

Shiitake mushrooms are able to help macrophage cells achieve this activated profile.

The cardiovascular benefits of shiitake mushrooms have been documented in three basic areas of research. The first of these areas is cholesterol reduction. d-Eritadenine (also called lentinacin, or lentsine, and sometimes abbreviated as DEA) is one of the most unusual, naturally occurring nutrients in shiitake mushrooms that has repeatedly been shown to help lower total blood cholesterol. Shiitake mushrooms can help protect us against cardiovascular diseases (including atherosclerosis) by preventing excessive immune cells binding to the lining of our blood vessels. Lastly, they are great antioxidant support. Chronic oxidative stress in our cardiovascular system is a critical factor of clogged arteries and other blood vessel problems. One of the best ways to reduce oxidative stress is the consumption of a diet rich in antioxidant nutrients. Shiitake mushrooms are a very good source of three key antioxidant minerals: manganese, selenium, and zinc.

On top of all these health benefits, shiitake mushrooms are wonderfully tasty and versatile. Anytime a recipe calls for a mushroom, use shiitake. Its meaty texture makes it a healthier alternative to the portabello mushroom. It may be more expensive, but that's because it has more nutritive value. And isn't your body worth it?

33. THE DEVIL'S TONGUE

Quintessential Japanese foods that help you lose weight are konnyaku and shirataki.

Actually, both konnyaku and shirataki come from plant stem of the konnyaku or konjac plant - also known as the Devil's Tongue plant due to its ugly look. Ironically, konnyaku is abundant in ceramide, an important moisturizing factor for skin beauty.

Konnyaku is used in traditional Japanese dishes such as "oden", a flavorful vegetable stew. Shirataki is just a long, thin noodle form of konnyaku, and is used in dishes such as sukiyaki.

Konnyaku and shirataki have almost zero calories. (No wonder, since their content is mostly water.) They also contain a soluble fiber called glucomannan which absorbs several times its weight in water, forming a gel in the stomach. This gel makes you feel full, slowing the digestion of fats. It's extremely effective in helping prevent or relieve constipation, and makes konnyaku a powerful weight loss food.

When I was teenager, I went on an extreme diet, by eating excessive amounts of konnyaku every day for a month. Obviously eating the same food excessively is stupid, but I was ignorant at that time. Anyway, while I lost a lot of weight that month, I finally tired of konnyaku and gained back the weight I had lost. Moderation is key.

Raw or canned konnyaku and shirataki can be found in most Asian supermarkets. Alternatively, "Tofu Shirataki" or "Noodle Tofu", sold by House Foods America in American supermarkets, is made from combining konnyaku with tofu. As such, it's a bit higher in calories than pure konnyaku, but still low enough in calories and rich in protein.

Shirataki noodles have been getting some attention as an alternative to pasta. As shirataki is flavorless, try replacing only 20% to 50% of your pasta to start, until you get used to its unique texture.

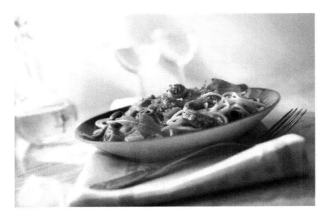

34. SOBA, THE SKINNY CARB

While the Japanese love Italian pasta too, their favorite carbohydrate is SOBA, buckwheat noodles, which happens to be perfect for weight loss.

Made from buckwheat and about the size of spaghetti, soba noodles can be served hot or cold. In Japan, New Year's Eve is traditionally celebrated with a bowl of hot soba noodles, called toshikoshi soba, which roughly means "end the old year and enter the new year" soba noodles. Soba symbolizes healthy happiness in a thin but long life. Throughout the year, you will find soba kiosks wherever you go and office workers, called "salary men" in Japan, noisily eat soba while standing. The slurping indicates enjoyment of the delicious soba, not a lack of manners.

These days, dried soba noodles can be readily found at gourmet grocery stores, oriental markets and even mainstream supermarkets. Made from healthy buckwheat, soba noodles have many nutritional and weight loss benefits.

A single 1 cup serving of cooked soba noodles has 113 calories and 24.4 g of carbs, compared to approximately 221 calories and 43.2 g of carbs in cooked spaghetti noodles.

Rutin in buckwheat strengthens capillaries and thus helps people suffering from arteriosclerosis and high blood pressure. Rutin helps stabilize Vitamin C, which produces collagen and prevents age spots. Buckwheat also contains choline which assists with increasing metabolism and decreasing fat accumulation; magnesium which helps contribute to your cardiovascular health by lowering your blood pressure and cholesterol levels; and is high in flavonoids, those antioxidants that protect your levels of good cholesterol from free radicals. The high fiber content of buckwheat also promotes regular bowel movements and prevents the bloating and intestinal back up that can cause temporary weight gain.

Now that you're convinced of the benefits of this superfood, here's a super easy soba recipe:

1. Cook soba noodles as directed. (To make them firm, rinse them with really cold water as soon as possible after cooking in hot water.)
2. Prepare your favorite vegetables.
3. Combine the noodles and the vegetables, and add sesame dressing to taste.

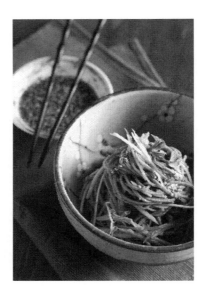

35. JAPANESE RICE CRACKERS

A favorite munchie of mine is the Japanese rice cracker, which makes for a healthy snack, especially when compared to high-calorie cookies, cakes and candy. Japanese rice crackers are usually thin and light with higher nutritional values than the sweet stuff.

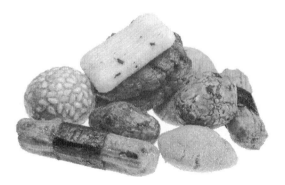

Rice crackers are generally made with rice, vegetable oil, and soy sauce (consisting of water, soybeans, wheat and salt). The salt and vegetable oil bring the healthy factor down a notch, but otherwise rice crackers don't contain excessively unhealthy ingredients like cholesterol and fat. They generally have no cholesterol, and a 21 g serving of two rice crackers has between 1 and 5 g of fat, depending on the brand. Even the salt content of a single rice cracker serving still remains at 100 mg or below, with sugar ranging between 1 and 5 g.

Rice crackers also contain between 1 and 4 g of protein, and 13 to 25 g of carbohydrates. Rice crackers may contain some iron and potassium, depending on the brand. A single serving of rice crackers has between 100 and 130 calories, a healthy number of calories for a snack, whereas a single serving of 15 potato chips can contain 150 calories and 10 g of fat. A single serving of five Saltines is lower in calories than Japanese rice crackers, with (60 versus at least 100 calories), but it's also higher in sodium, with (190 mg versus 25 to 100 mg).

Japanese rice crackers get their crispiness and delicious flavor from grilling, not deep-frying. The variety of rice cracker flavors available offers you a healthier complement to your cheese tray than traditional crackers. And they are way better than digging into a bag of potato chips when you have that sudden snack craving. I always carry a small bag of rice crackers with me for that very reason.

TIPS FOR THINGS YOU
DON'T USUALLY THINK ABOUT

36. YOUR PELVIS, THE KEY TO FITNESS

Sounds odd, I know...but to understand the impact of a strong, balanced pelvis on your body, you need to take a look at how this basin-shaped structure at the base of the spinal column actually works.

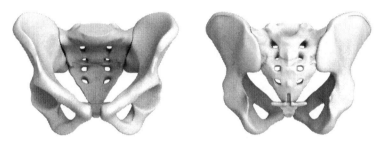

Front and back views of the pelvis

Think of the pelvis as the bottom half of a spinning top; if it's not pointing straight up and down, there is no way—no matter how much momentum you give it—that the top will spin. Simply put: if it's off balance, you might be, too.

Just like that spinning top, the pelvis--a soft, bony structure--runs the show. It's the foundation of your whole body, the bridge that connects your upper and lower half, and a cradle for your internal organs and genitalia. Americans are focusing on the core these days, and the pelvis is the foundation of core. Training it, balancing it, and being kind to it results in a long, tall, efficiently working body. Here are five solid reasons to perfect your pelvis...

- **You'll lose weight.** When your pelvis is perfectly placed, your internal organs line up, too. This means your circulation and metabolism become more efficient, and your transmitter nerves have a direct line to the appetite center, signaling the brain when you're full.

- **Your hormonal organs will function at an optimal level.** When the pelvis is in correct alignment, your ovaries and uterus are protected, reducing your chances of having irregular periods, menstrual pain, or significant menopausal symptoms.

- **You'll have a well-proportioned figure.** The pelvis is a soft, mobile structure, which is why it widens or opens to permit the birth of a baby, and can throw you off-kilter as a result. In its proper, closed position, the pelvis forces your butt, thigh, calf, and belly muscles to work in tandem, so no one area becomes overly bulky.

- **Back pain is diminished.** When the pelvis is correctly lined up, your core ab muscles spring into action, reducing the reliance on your back, and any resulting pain and injury that goes along with it.

- **Constipation won't be an issue.** Your pelvis protects the intestines and bladder, shielding them from the pressure of internal organs, which can result in irregular bowel movements.

Convinced? Good! Now let me show you how to whip that pelvis into shape....

- **Practice good posture, standing or sitting.**

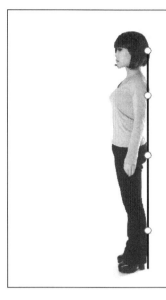

When you stand, align your body correctly; you can do so by standing against a wall. Ideally, your head, shoulder blades, butt, calves, and heels are all touching the wall, and you could draw a straight line from your head to your toes, much like a puppet on a string.

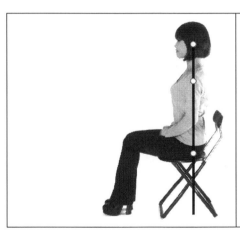

The basic is the same as when you are standing, but your upper back and thighs are at a 90 degree angle while sitting. Imagine placing your head weight on your anus, so that you don't hunch over too much, especially when at the computer.

- **Do the "model walk".** (More on that in the next chapter.)

- **Train your ab muscles.** They help support and stabilize the pelvis, enabling it to stay in a perfect position.

- **Vary the hands you use for carrying things.** If you're right-handed, you'll probably have to make a concerted effort to carry things in your left, too; but doing so will keep you balanced.

- **Don't cross your legs when seated.** It throws the works off-kilter. If you cannot sit without crossing your legs, that's a sign that your pelvis is open and distorted, as body tries to stabilize by crossing legs.

- **Sleep on your back.** Think about it: one-third of your day is spent in a reclining position...make sure it's one that's kind to your pelvis. I actually like sleeping with a travel neck-roll pillow (even at home), because it helps me stay on my back throughout the night.

37. LOOK YOUNGER WITH THE HIGH-FASHION WALK

People always associate "the walk" with high-fashion runway shows, but when you get right down to it, a model's walk isn't just for models...it's for anyone who wants to look and be lean, long, and young, while avoiding some serious knee and back pain. Historically, the Japanese aren't the best people to emulate for a good gait, given that we've been saddled with kimonos and zori (slippers), known to restrict proper leg movement.

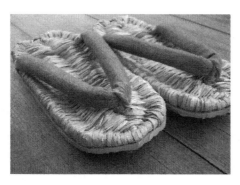

But Western clothes (and no, I'm not talking about boots and cowboy hats here) allow the kind of efficient stride that results in head-to-toe benefits: good posture; strong ab muscles; long legs; a tight butt; firm, lifted breasts; and a toned, taut back. I'll let you in on another secret: I've personally gained an inch in the height department, because walking correctly adjusts posture, as opposed to the "shrinkage" many people experience as they age.

I truly believe in a mind/body connection, and posture is a key component there, too. When I stand up straight, open my chest, and gaze upwards, I find myself feeling happier, less depressed, and more optimistic about life. It may be a bit of the "which came first; the chicken or the egg?" scenario, but when you walk "up", you feel "up", and vice versa.

Want to walk the walk? A picture (or five!) is worth a thousand words:

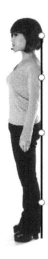

1. (See photo left): Before you take a single step, you have to align your body correctly; you can do so by standing against a wall. Ideally, your head, shoulder blades, butt, calves, and heels are all touching the wall, and you could draw a straight line from your head to your toes, much like a puppet on a string.

2. Slip your hand into the small of your back--you should be able to fit no more than one hand in that space. Able to make a fist? That means you've got more curvature (a.k.a. "sway back") than you need, and it's time for an adjustment: simply shift your pelvis forward, allowing your weight to settle into your buttocks slightly. Now, try the hand trick again; the space should be smaller.

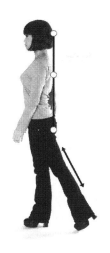

3. It's time to start moving: straighten and stretch out whichever leg you'd like to start on, making sure your heel—not your toe—touches the ground first.

4. (See photo left): Now focus on the opposite leg, making sure it, too, is outstretched behind you. Use its power to propel you forward, feeling your butt tighten as your back leg kicks out. After a quick posture check to make sure your breasts, abs, and front leg are still in line, you can allow your weight to settle evenly into your abs and both legs.

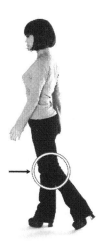

5. Next step (literally): bend your back leg, allowing one knee to gently graze the other, creating a triangle shape in that space between the two. Touching those knees together forces you to rely on your inner-thigh muscles, which in turn helps avoid that bulky quad look people get from overworking the front of their thighs.

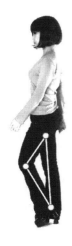

6.   Move your leg forward and create another triangle in the front.

Once you've nailed the proper gait, practice taking longer strides, which maximizes muscle use and helps increase your metabolism

38. ANTI-AGING BREAST CARE

It's been called everything from "back fat" to "bra fat" to "spillover" to "rolls", but the skin that bulges out from your underarms, sides, and back is actually considered to be a part of your breasts.

Scientifically speaking, it's known as Cooper's ligaments, and is comprised of connective tissue that helps maintain the structural integrity of your breasts and surrounding areas. With the same elasticity you would find in a rubber band, these ligaments are designed to stretch; and just like a rubber band, they can stretch too much...to a point where they are too weak to return to their original size and shape.

And this is why it's critical to be fitted with a supportive bra, and learn exactly how to wear it. If you end up with one that's too small, you'll risk damaging delicate breast tissue due to being smashed up against side wires. Wear one in the wrong position, and you'll reveal excess skin that gives you an unflattering—even aging—look. (Quick tip: I actually take my new bras to the tailor, altering them so that my breasts are perfectly aligned without any sag. Considering that a good-quality bra can cost upwards of $60, it's a worthwhile investment.)

How to Properly Fit Into Your Bra

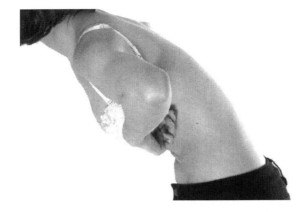

1. Lean forward 45 degrees and bring the bra cups up to your breasts.

2. While in this position, fasten the hooks so your breasts are actually placed in the cups correctly.

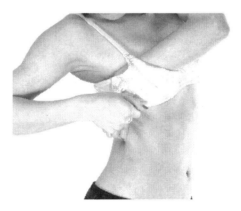

3. Return to an upward position, and bend 45 degrees to the right, gently tucking excess skin from your back, sides, and underarms into the bra. Repeat this process on the left side.

4. Now stand up straight and check the position of your bra in a mirror. Adjust the straps as close to your underarms as comfortably possible, making sure the cups are lying flat against your breasts with no visible gaps.

5. Pull the back band of the bra downward a bit, maximizing the support of your breasts.

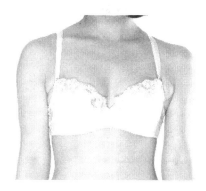

Incorrect fit

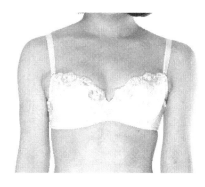

Correct fit

Of course, once you've got the fit down right, you may want to focus on fashion: fortunately, there are plenty of gorgeous bras on the market, making them a virtual accessory unto themselves. (Believe it or not, in Japan, bras are even marketed to a male clientele, who appreciate the feminine flair of fine lingerie. Think I'm kidding? I'm not!)

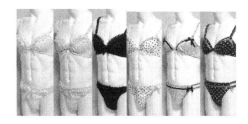

39. AGING BODY ODOR:
HOW TO FIGHT THE "FRAGRANCE"

Believe it or not, body odor changes with age. During your skin's natural maturation phase, oxidized fatty acids from the sebaceous glands release an odor substance known as "Nonenal", a phenomenon first discovered by researchers at the Japanese cosmetics company, Shiseido. "It's scientifically proven that body odor changes with age. As skin matures, its natural antioxidant defenses decrease, resulting in Nonenal, an odor phenomenon", says Dr. Kato, advising anti-aging specialist of Mirai Clinical. Unlike conventional body odor caused by the build-up of bacteria (from a sweaty workout, say), Nonenal cannot be eliminated by simply sudsing up with regular soap and water. It is not the type of body odor which regular soaps can deodorize.

While it affects both men and women, menopause actually plays a role in revving up the process. Let me explain how it occurs.

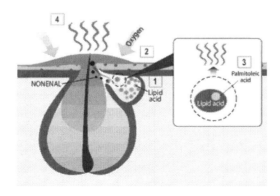

1. During menopause, as estrogen levels decrease, male hormone ratios are increased. This process results in more lipid acid (fatty acid) production in the sebaceous gland.

2. At the same time, as skin matures, its natural antioxidant protection decreases.

3. Palmitoleic acid in lipid acid therefore is oxidized.

4. This results in the production of an unsaturated aldehyde, Nonenal.

Hot flashes and night sweats during menopause cause excessive perspiration and increased fatty acids, also resulting in Nonenal. In addition, stress can also exacerbate the production of Nonenal.

The Japanese, who are known to be clean fanatics, have been particularly plugged in to the Nonenal phenomenon, and take great pains to combat its resulting unpleasant, greasy-like smell. In fact, for some, like the male commuters on packed Tokyo trains (who have to raise their arms and hold onto ceiling rails to avoid inadvertently "groping" female passengers), reducing Nonenal odor is imperative. You can do that by simply following a healthy lifestyle as much as possible which includes exercising, getting plenty of rest, avoiding stress and smoking, drinking alcoholic beverages in moderation, and eating a really clean diet. Here at Mirai Clinical, we've taken further steps to help people deal with the problem by incorporating natural, odor-fighting ingredients, such as Japanese persimmon extract (the Japanese have used it for centuries to combat BO) and purified green tea, into our Purifying Body Wash, Deodorizing Persimmon Bar, and Purifying Body Spritzer. These natural ingredients literally eliminate odor instantly, and I particularly recommend them to anyone over the age of 40.

40. ANTI-AGING TOILET TRAINING

They say multi-tasking is the way of the world these days, so I'm going to get a bit graphic and let you in on an exercise maneuver that the Japanese have historically used when going to the bathroom:

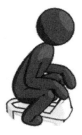

Unlike Western-style toilets (in which you sit down on the commode), Japanese traditional toileting has often been done in a squat position that forces you to engage your thigh muscles, which—just like when you train your quads in the gym—helps strengthen your legs and rev up your metabolism.

Though many urban Japanese bathrooms are now modernized with Western-style toilets, you can still borrow the original technique by rising ever so slightly off the seat, and holding this position as long as possible.

While you're at it, practice your Kegel exercises, which strengthen your pelvic floor (and the muscles that control urine flow), tighten your tush, improve sexual satisfaction, and prevent light bladder leakage. It's simple: as you're urinating, stop the flow for a few seconds, then release and repeat. Between the squats and the Kegels, you're basically in training mode some 2,000 extra times a year!

41. THE POOP TEST

Ever since I moved to the United States, I've had the distinct impression that the Japanese are more comfortable with their bodily functions, which---at the risk of sounding like a Kindergartener---include peeing, pooping, farting, and burping. I mean, when you think about it, these are simply physical "jobs" that every single body in the entire world is designed to do. The Japanese have actually capitalized on these functions by inventing high-tech toilets with built-in bidets (such as TOTO which include customizable spray and power angles); advanced features that measure your weight, blood pressure, and body temperature; music options; and even technology that relays information about your urine directly to your doctor (no plastic cup needed!).

With "intestinal beauty" being a big buzzword in Japan these days, it might not surprise you to hear that some of the Japanese actually keep a diary of their bowel movements to help them monitor their own level of health. Young students are taught to understand the importance of the intestinal process, and how to maintain it in their science classes. And—I'm totally serious here—there's actually a beauty contest in which contestants compete for perfect poop. (Don't worry, the judges look clinically at their insides, not their toilet water!)

If you can step away from the cultural squeamishness for a minute and think of your bowel movements as your own, personal healthcare report, you'll realize you actually have a tool that delivers everything from information about what foods you've digested to your general well being. What goes in (hopefully, wise and nutritious food choices) must come out—a natural detoxification process that allows your cells to rejuvenate on a daily basis. Become constipated, and you're actually putting the brakes on your body's own method of eliminating 75 percent of the toxins and waste products in your body to make room for new, healthful nutrients. (Your detox is comprised of as much as 75% from bowel movements, 20% from urine and 5% from hair, nails, and sweat.) You'll also make yourself vulnerable to the harmful bacteria that leads to poor metabolism, a diminished immune system, skin breakouts, body odor, and even, in some cases, colon cancer. Fortunately, avoiding constipation is—for most people—a matter of four simple steps:

1. Eat plenty of fiber-rich foods, such as whole grains, fruits, and cruciferous vegetables.
2. Drink water when you wake up, and continue your daily intake of clear fluids, such as water, green tea and fruit juices.
3. Get enough exercise.
4. Visit the restroom as soon as you feel the urge to go. Once you're on the toilet, allow yourself to relax in order to produce a healthy bowel movement.

When I spend time in Japan, because of the healthier Japanese diet, I'm always surprised how my healthy diet is reflected in my bowel movements. Let me show you exactly what I mean....okay, here's Poop 101:

The Perfect Poop:

- Shaped like a banana, and comes out quickly and smoothly.
- The same texture as a banana—not too hard, not too soft. 80% is water.
- Golden in color.
- It floats in the water (because it contains enough fiber).
- Not overly smelly.
- Leaves you with a clean wipe (nothing, or almost nothing, on the toilet paper).
- Has the heft of two-to-four bananas per day.

The Aging Ploppy Poop:

- Skinny-looking.
- The result of insufficient calories or weak ab muscles.
- Dark-reddish-brown to black in color.
- Is produced in several pieces.
- Very smelly.
- Texture like an ink tube.

The fix: Increase your fiber intake; eat probiotic yogurt; train your ab muscles.

The Muddy Poop:

* Has the texture of mud.
* Is dark-brown or black in color.
* Very smelly.
* Liquid-y because of its high water content (about 88%).

The fix: Increase your fiber intake; get plenty of rest and relaxation; if it continues more than a few days, consult your doctor.

The Watery Poop (aka, Diarrhea):

* Sudden urge to move bowels that results in pure liquid (about 90% water).
* Brown in color.
* Very smelly.
* Equivalent in measurement to two-to-three cups of coffee.
* Can signify that the mucus membrane lining of the colon is irritated.

The fix: Avoid stress and overeating; avoid spicy foods; warm your body temperature; if it continues for more than a day or two, consult your doctor.

The Combo Confused Poop:

* A combination of hard and watery stools.
* Light brown in color.
* Equivalent in measurement to one-to-two cups of coffee.
* Can be smelly or not.

The fix: Avoid stress, as this type of stool can be attributed to Irritable Bowel Syndrome; eat a balanced diet; relax in a warm tub.

The Rabbit Poop (aka, Constipation):

* Hard, small "pebbles".
* Brown to dark-reddish-brown in color.
* Extremely smelly.
* A distended abdomen caused by sluggish bowels.
* Very little water content (60% water)

The fix: Increase fiber intake; avoid resisting the urge to move your bowels; drink plenty of water.

WHEN LESS IS MORE

42. LAUGHTER FOR OPTIMAL HEALTH

Laughter is the easiest, no-cost therapy for anti-aging and optimal health.

There are sixty trillion cells in our body and most of them can be rejuvenated. Sometimes our bodies produce cancer cells, often up to 5,000 cancer cells every day, which are naturally destroyed by your healthy white blood cells. Smoking, excessive alcohol consumption, stress, MSG or junk foods can lower your natural resistance. To boost your natural immunity, just laugh!

As we age, our opportunities to laugh tend to decrease. So, it's important to try to enjoy such opportunities.

Laughter boosts the immune system. Laughter decreases stress hormones and increases immune cells and infection-fighting antibodies, thus improving your resistance to disease. Laughter improves blood circulation and trains your mouth muscles, perfect for anti-aging face care. Laughter releases pain, physically and emotionally. It relieves anxiety. One cannot laugh and be afraid simultaneously; it's physically impossible. Laughter also shrinks the source and size of our fears. It reduces aggression and conflict. People laughing are unable to hold each other at sword point. It is part of the body's biological drug store.

Hospitals actually provide laughter therapy, but of course healthy people can get benefits, too.

Laughter is universal. Everybody can laugh. Human beings are born with the gift of laughter. A sense of humor is not necessary to laugh. Laughter decreases feelings of isolation. Laughter allows us to bond with other people and ease our loneliness. Laughter creates laughter; it's contagious. Allowing laughter to swell into a movement across the land would reduce our growing anger and violence in the long term. It even allows us to be creative and to work harder but more comfortably.

Last but not least, it's just fun. It gives us back our playfulness, a characteristic of all mankind.

In Japan, Laughter Yoga is a trend now. Companies practice laughter yoga in the morning, which has been found to increase work efficiency. Laughter Yoga combines Unconditional Laughter with Yogic Breathing. Anyone can Laugh for No Reason, without relying on humor, jokes or comedy. Laughter is simulated as a body exercise in a group; with eye contact and childlike playfulness; it soon turns into real and contagious laughter. The concept of Laughter Yoga was born in India and is based on a scientific fact that the body cannot differentiate between fake and real laughter, and one gets the same physiological and psychological benefits either way. Laughter Yoga was practiced even in shelters after the earthquake and tsunami in Japan.

When in doubt, just laugh.

43. LIFE CLEANSE

We started this book looking to the past, learning from centuries-old Japanese practices. Now, let's look to the future.

A new word has been added to the Japanese vocabulary, "Dansyari". Directly translated, it means "life cleaning", or:

Dan: Say 'no' to unnecessary things. When you are invited to a party which you do not want to attend but feel you have to, even if you won't enjoy yourself, just say no. This is quite revolutionary in Japan, as Japanese people in general cannot say "no".

Sya: Throw away unnecessary things. Physical clutter creates mental clutter. You keep an old cap because a good friend gave it to you, but you never wear it. This cap, then, is a waste of space, an obstruction in your mind, and creates guilt from not wearing it. So, if you have not used it in a year, give it away or throw it away even if it's an expensive item. In Japan, there is a concept called "mottainai" which means feeling sorry for not using something because it's a waste. If you have new shirt you've never worn, that's "mottainai".

Ri: Stop obsessing about unnecessary things. Use only what you need. Eat only what you need. Do only what you need to. Say only what you need to say.

As Japan is a small country with small homes, dansyari fits neatly into Japanese households. But it's not just for removing clutter, but also for cleaning up your life. Japan is experiencing a new boom in people reading books, taking seminars, and participating in social activities, in order to learn more about dansyari.

Less Is More.

ABOUT THE AUTHOR

Born and raised on Japan's northernmost island, Hokkaido, renowned for its clean air, water, and lifestyle, Koko Hayashi has cultivated a life-long interest in natural treatments and skin care. After receiving an Undergraduate degree from Sapporo University and an MBA at the Chinese University of Hong Kong, she successfully completed the prestigious CIDESCO degree, the internationally respected aesthetic license requiring a deep understanding of the human body and its functions. As an expert on Japanese anti-aging philosophy and practices, she is dedicated to improving people's quality of life, and is now introducing her knowledge to the world.

Made in the USA
Monee, IL
05 February 2020

21332050R00079